The Nurse's Clinical Guide to Addiction and Recovery

A Practical Toolkit for Withdrawal Management, MAT, and Trauma-Informed Care

I0140488

Theo Seki

ISBN: 978-1-7641941-8-1

Isohan Publishing

Table of Contents

Chapter 1: The Modern Understanding of Addiction 1

Chapter 2: The Pharmacopeia of Substance Use 9

Chapter 3: Screening, Brief Intervention, and Referral to Treatment (SBIRT) 18

Chapter 4: Motivational Interviewing (MI) 28

Chapter 5: Managing Withdrawal 36

Chapter 6: Medication-Assisted Treatment (MAT)........................... 43

Chapter 7: Addressing Co-Occurring Disorders.................................. 48

Chapter 8: Deconstructing Stigma and Bias in Healthcare 53

Chapter 9: Trauma-Informed Care 58

Chapter 10: The Harm Reduction Philosophy in Practice 63

Chapter 11: Case Studies from the Front Lines.................................. 69

Appendix: The Nurse's Quick-Reference Toolkit 77

References 82

Chapter 1: The Modern Understanding of Addiction

Beyond a Moral Failing

It is a scenario as old as nursing itself. You have a patient—let's call him Mr. Gable—in bed four, recovering from a complicated abdominal surgery. His pain is poorly controlled, he's pressing the PCA pump button with a frantic regularity that sets your teeth on edge, and his chart contains the neatly coded history: "Opioid Use Disorder." The morning report from the off-going nurse was laced with sighs and eye-rolls. "Good luck with bed four," she said, "He's a real clock-watcher." In that moment, a cascade of judgments and assumptions can so easily begin, painting a picture of a person who is manipulative, weak-willed, or simply seeking a high. This chapter is about dismantling that picture. It is about replacing the worn-out, stigmatizing frame of a moral failing with the scientifically grounded and clinically useful framework of a complex brain condition. To care for Mr. Gable effectively, and for the millions like him, we must first fundamentally shift our understanding.

From Moral Weakness to a Brain Condition

For centuries, societies have viewed substance dependence through a lens of morality. A person who could not control their use of alcohol or other drugs was considered weak, sinful, or constitutionally flawed. This perspective—while deeply ingrained in our culture—is clinically useless and demonstrably false. It creates shame, drives people away from care, and prevents us from applying effective, evidence-based interventions.

The modern understanding, grounded in decades of neurobiological and psychological research, reframes addiction as a **biopsychosocial condition**. Let's break that down, because it's more than just a piece of academic jargon; it is the foundation of compassionate and effective nursing care.

- **Bio:** This refers to the brain and body. It encompasses a person's genetic predispositions—some individuals are simply more genetically susceptible to developing a substance use disorder than others—and, most importantly, the profound changes that substances make to the brain's structure and function.

- **Psycho:** This involves an individual's unique psychological landscape. Factors like a history of trauma, co-occurring mental health conditions (like depression or anxiety), learned behaviors, and even a person's core beliefs about themselves and the world can contribute to the development and maintenance of a substance use disorder.

- **Social:** A person does not exist in a vacuum. Their social environment—including family relationships, community support (or lack thereof), socioeconomic status, cultural norms, and exposure to stress and violence—plays a powerful role.

Thinking in this way moves us from asking, "What is wrong with you?" to asking the far more productive question, "What has happened to you?" It allows us to see the whole person, not just the behavior that is causing the immediate problem.

The Brain on Drugs: A Primer for Nurses

You do not need a Ph.D. in neuroscience to understand the basics of what happens in the brain. At its heart, addiction is a disorder of the brain's reward system—a primitive, powerful set of circuits designed to ensure our survival by encouraging life-sustaining behaviors like eating and procreating.

1. **The Reward Pathway:** When we do something enjoyable, a part of the brain called the ventral tegmental area (VTA) releases a neurotransmitter called **dopamine** into another area, the nucleus accumbens. You can think of dopamine as the "Go!" signal or the "Do that again!" chemical. It tells the brain that whatever just happened was good and should be repeated.

2. **The Substance Hijacking:** Drugs of misuse do not just tap into this system; they hijack it. They cause a flood of dopamine

that is far more intense and reliable than any natural reward. For example, a substance like cocaine can increase dopamine levels to a degree that dwarfs the response from eating a good meal or having a pleasant social interaction. This creates an incredibly powerful—and artificial—"Go!" signal.

3. **The Development of Craving:** The brain, always trying to maintain balance, adapts to this repeated, overwhelming dopamine surge. It may start producing less dopamine on its own or reduce the number of dopamine receptors. The result? The person's natural reward system is blunted. Things that used to bring pleasure no longer do. The only thing that can make them feel good—or even just feel "normal"—is the substance. This is the neurobiological root of craving: the brain is sending a desperate signal that it needs the substance to restore its chemical equilibrium.

4. **The "Hungry Ghost" Within:** Dr. Gabor Maté, a physician who has written extensively on addiction, uses a powerful metaphor from Buddhist cosmology to describe this state: the "hungry ghost" [1]. This is a creature with a massive, empty stomach and a pinhole mouth. It is constantly starving, driven by an insatiable hunger, but can never, ever get enough to feel full. This is a perfect analogy for the experience of craving. It is not a simple desire; it is a profound, gnawing emptiness and a desperate, compulsive drive to fill it, even when the person knows it will only bring more suffering. It is a state of profound internal distress.

This process is a form of **neuroplasticity**—the brain's ability to change and rewire itself. Unfortunately, in this case, it has rewired itself around the substance. The good news, however, is that neuroplasticity works both ways. With time, treatment, and support, the brain can and does begin to heal and form new, healthier pathways. That is the biological basis of recovery.

The Critical Importance of Language

3

Before we proceed any further, we must address the tools of our trade—our words. The language we use has a direct impact on the care we provide. Stigmatizing language reinforces negative stereotypes and creates barriers between us and our patients. Person-centered language, on the other hand, promotes dignity and builds the therapeutic alliance that is so essential for healing.

Therefore, throughout this book and in your practice, you must commit to a new vocabulary.

- Instead of "addict" or "abuser," say **"a person with a substance use disorder."**

- Instead of "clean" or "dirty" urine, say **"the urine drug screen was negative"** or **"positive for substances."**

- Instead of "drug habit," say **"substance use disorder"** or **"risky substance use."**

- Instead of "relapse," which implies failure, consider using **"a return to use"** or **"a recurrence of symptoms."**

This is not about being "politically correct." It is about being clinically precise and demonstrating respect. You would not call a patient in bed five a "diabetic"; you would say she is "a person with diabetes." We must afford the same dignity to people with substance use disorders.

Case Examples in Practice

Case Example 1: Mr. Henderson, the Post-Surgical Patient

Mr. Henderson is a 55-year-old man on his third day post-op after a knee replacement. His medical history includes a "heroin use disorder, in remission." He is reporting pain of 9/10 and is requesting pain medication an hour before it is due. The nurse, feeling frustrated, initially thinks, "He's just drug-seeking."

- **Applying the Biopsychosocial Model:** Instead of focusing solely on the behavior, the nurse considers the full picture.

  - **Bio:** She knows that Mr. Henderson's long-term opioid use has likely altered his brain's reward and pain pathways, making him more sensitive to pain (a condition known as hyperalgesia) and blunting his response to the prescribed opioid medication. His brain is not processing pain or relief in the same way as a person without his history.

  - **Psycho:** She considers the immense anxiety Mr. Henderson must be feeling. He is in legitimate, severe pain, but he knows how his request is perceived. He is terrified of being undertreated and equally terrified of a recurrence of his substance use disorder.

  - **Social:** He is alone in the hospital, away from his usual support systems. He feels judged by the staff, which increases his stress and, in turn, his perception of pain.

- **Intervention:** The nurse changes her approach. She sits with Mr. Henderson and says, "It sounds like you are in a tremendous amount of pain. This must be incredibly difficult, especially with your history. Let's work together on a better plan." By acknowledging his reality and using non-judgmental language, she builds trust. They discuss non-pharmacological options like ice and repositioning, and she consults with the medical team about a multimodal pain management plan that might be more effective than opioids alone.

Case Example 2: Maria, the Clinic Patient

Maria is a 28-year-old woman who comes to a primary care clinic for a routine check-up. During the screening, she admits to drinking "a bottle of wine or so" most nights to "take the edge off." The nurse could easily label this a "bad habit" and move on.

- **Applying the Biopsychosocial Model:** The nurse decides to ask more questions.

5

- **Psycho:** She learns that Maria has a history of significant childhood trauma and struggles with severe anxiety. The alcohol is not for fun; it is a form of self-medication to quiet the intrusive thoughts and panic she experiences. She is using alcohol to manage an underlying, untreated psychological wound.

- **Social:** Maria recently lost her job and is feeling isolated from her friends. The nightly drinking has become her primary coping mechanism and her main companion.

- **Intervention:** Using person-first language, the nurse says, "It sounds like you've been through a lot, and you've found something that helps you get through the day. Thank you for trusting me enough to share that." She then gently explains how alcohol, while seeming to help in the short term, can actually worsen anxiety over time. She offers a referral to a therapist who specializes in trauma and discusses the possibility of medications that could treat Maria's anxiety more safely and effectively. The conversation is about providing support, not passing judgment.

Case Example 3: David, the Emergency Department Patient

David, 19, is brought to the Emergency Department by paramedics after being found unresponsive. He has pinpoint pupils and slow, shallow breathing. The team administers naloxone, and he awakens abruptly, disoriented and agitated. A staff member mutters, "Another overdose."

- **Applying the Biopsychosocial Model:** The primary nurse quiets the room and focuses on David.

  - **Bio:** Her immediate priority is his physiological state—his breathing, his oxygen saturation, his neurological status. She understands his agitation is a direct result of the naloxone violently displacing opioids from the receptors in his brain, throwing him into sudden,

6

severe withdrawal. It is a physiological reaction, not a character flaw.

- ○ **Psycho:** She speaks to him in a calm, reassuring voice. "David, you're in the hospital. You're safe. We gave you a medicine to help you breathe." She knows he is likely feeling terrified and deeply ashamed.

- **Intervention:** Instead of lecturing him, she provides comfort—a warm blanket, a quiet space once he is stable. Once he is calmer, she approaches him not with accusations, but with an offer of help. "That was really scary. We have people here who can talk to you about what happened and help you find ways to stay safe. Would you be open to speaking with one of them?" This approach respects his autonomy and opens the door for a referral to treatment, rather than simply discharging him back to the same circumstances.

Key Takeaways for Your Practice

- Substance use disorder is a biopsychosocial condition, not a moral failing. Your approach to care must reflect this understanding.

- The brain's reward system is hijacked by substances, leading to profound changes in brain chemistry and function that drive craving and compulsive use.

- The language you use matters immensely. Adopt person-first language to reduce stigma and build therapeutic relationships.

- Always look beyond the behavior to understand the person and the complex factors contributing to their substance use.

Having established this foundational understanding of *why* individuals develop substance use disorders, we must now turn our attention to the practical matter of *what* they are using. A proficient nurse must be able to recognize the signs and symptoms associated with the major classes of substances to provide safe and effective care.

Chapter 2: The Pharmacopeia of Substance Use

What Nurses Need to Know

In the fast-paced and often chaotic world of clinical nursing, there is rarely time for leisurely review. When a patient arrives in the emergency department with a dangerously slow heart rate and pinpoint pupils, or when a patient on a medical-surgical floor suddenly becomes tremulous and hypertensive, you need to recognize the potential cause and act swiftly. This chapter is designed to be your quick-reference guide to the major classes of substances you will encounter. It is not an exhaustive pharmacology textbook—it is a field guide. We will focus on what you need to know at the bedside: how to spot intoxication, what to expect during withdrawal, and the key risks to anticipate.

Opioids

Opioids are powerful pain relievers that act on opioid receptors in the brain, spinal cord, and other organs. This class includes everything from prescription medications to illicitly manufactured substances. Given the ongoing opioid crisis, this is a class of substances with which every nurse must be intimately familiar.

- **Common Street Names:** Heroin (smack, dope, H), Fentanyl (fent, fenty), prescription opioids like oxycodone (oxys, blues, 30s) and hydrocodone (vics, norcos). Be aware that illicitly manufactured pills are often pressed to look like legitimate pharmaceuticals but frequently contain lethal amounts of fentanyl.

- **Mechanism of Action:** Opioids bind to mu-opioid receptors in the brain, which produces feelings of euphoria and profound pain relief. Unfortunately, this action also suppresses the respiratory drive in the brainstem, which is the primary mechanism of overdose death.

- **Signs of Intoxication:** Think of the classic "opioid triad": **pinpoint pupils (miosis), respiratory depression** (slow, shallow breathing), and a **decreased level of consciousness**. Patients may appear sleepy, "nodding off," or completely unresponsive. You might also observe slurred speech, a slow heart rate, and low blood pressure.

- **Withdrawal Syndrome and Timeline:** While opioid withdrawal is intensely uncomfortable, it is not typically life-threatening in otherwise healthy individuals. The symptoms are often described as being like a severe case of the flu. The onset and duration depend on the specific opioid used (short-acting like heroin vs. long-acting like methadone).

  - **Early Symptoms (6-12 hours after last use for short-acting opioids):** Muscle aches, agitation, anxiety, watery eyes, runny nose, sweating, yawning.

  - **Late Symptoms (peaking around 72 hours):** Nausea, vomiting, diarrhea, abdominal cramping, goosebumps (piloerection—hence the term "cold turkey"), enlarged pupils, and intense cravings.

- **Long-Term Health Consequences:** Chronic constipation, risk of infectious diseases (HIV, Hepatitis C) from injection drug use, skin abscesses, and infection of the heart valves (endocarditis).

Alcohol

Alcohol (ethanol) is a central nervous system depressant and is one of the most widely used substances in the world. Its accessibility means you will see the effects of its use in every single clinical setting.

- **Mechanism of Action:** Alcohol enhances the effect of the inhibitory neurotransmitter GABA (gamma-aminobutyric acid) and suppresses the effect of the excitatory neurotransmitter glutamate. This is what causes the classic signs of intoxication—slurred speech, poor coordination, and sedation.

- **Signs of Intoxication:** The signs are familiar to most: slurred speech, impaired coordination (ataxia), unsteady gait, impaired judgment, and drowsiness. In severe cases, it can lead to respiratory depression, coma, and death.

- **Withdrawal Syndrome and Timeline:** Alcohol withdrawal is a medical emergency. The brain, accustomed to the constant depressant effect of alcohol, becomes massively overexcited when the alcohol is removed. This can be fatal. The timeline can vary, but a general guide is:

    o **6-12 hours:** Minor withdrawal symptoms begin. These include anxiety, insomnia, nausea, and tremors (the "shakes").

    o **12-24 hours:** Alcoholic hallucinosis may occur. This involves visual, auditory, or tactile hallucinations, but the patient is typically aware that they are hallucinating.

    o **24-48 hours:** Withdrawal seizures ("rum fits") can occur.

    o **48-72 hours (and beyond): Delirium Tremens (DTs)** may develop. This is the most severe form of withdrawal and is characterized by profound confusion, disorientation, agitation, fever, tachycardia, and hypertension. It carries a significant mortality rate if untreated.

- **Long-Term Health Consequences:** Liver disease (from fatty liver to cirrhosis), pancreatitis, gastritis and gastrointestinal bleeding, cardiomyopathy, peripheral neuropathy, and brain damage (Wernicke-Korsakoff syndrome).

Stimulants

This class of drugs does exactly what the name implies: it stimulates the central nervous system, leading to increased energy, alertness, and euphoria. This category includes both prescription medications and illicit substances.

- **Common Street Names:** Cocaine (coke, blow, snow), Crack Cocaine (rock), Methamphetamine (meth, crank, crystal, ice), prescription stimulants like amphetamine/dextroamphetamine (Adderall) and methylphenidate (Ritalin).

- **Mechanism of Action:** Stimulants work primarily by increasing the levels of dopamine and norepinephrine in the brain. This creates intense feelings of energy, focus, and pleasure.

- **Signs of Intoxication:** Think of a system in overdrive. You will see **dilated pupils (mydriasis)**, hyperactivity, talkativeness, and agitation. Physiologically, look for a high heart rate (tachycardia), high blood pressure (hypertension), and sweating. Patients may exhibit paranoia, panic, and in severe cases, psychosis with hallucinations and delusions.

- **Withdrawal Syndrome and Timeline:** Unlike alcohol or benzodiazepine withdrawal, stimulant withdrawal is not typically associated with major physical danger. However, it can be psychologically grueling. The main feature is the "crash."

    o **Symptoms:** Intense depression (sometimes with suicidal ideation), fatigue, increased need for sleep (hypersomnia), anxiety, and powerful cravings.

- **Long-Term Health Consequences:** For cocaine, cardiac complications are a major risk—myocardial infarction, arrhythmias, and cardiomyopathy. For methamphetamine, severe dental decay ("meth mouth"), skin sores from picking, and significant weight loss are common. All stimulants carry a risk of long-term psychiatric problems, including persistent psychosis.

Benzodiazepines

These are prescription medications typically used to treat anxiety, insomnia, and seizure disorders. Due to their sedative effects, they are frequently used non-medically.

- **Common Names:** Alprazolam (Xanax), Lorazepam (Ativan), Diazepam (Valium), Clonazepam (Klonopin). Street names often incorporate the brand name, like "xans" or "bars" for Xanax.

- **Mechanism of Action:** Like alcohol, benzodiazepines work by enhancing the effects of the inhibitory neurotransmitter GABA. This calms the nervous system.

- **Signs of Intoxication:** The presentation is very similar to alcohol intoxication: drowsiness, confusion, slurred speech, poor coordination, and memory problems. When combined with other depressants like alcohol or opioids, the risk of life-threatening respiratory depression is extremely high.

- **Withdrawal Syndrome and Timeline: Benzodiazepine withdrawal can be life-threatening and should never be done abruptly.** The symptoms are a mirror image of the drug's effects: intense anxiety, insomnia, restlessness, and tremors. Like alcohol withdrawal, it can also lead to seizures. The withdrawal from long-acting benzodiazepines like diazepam can be delayed and prolonged for weeks or even months.

- **Long-Term Health Consequences:** Cognitive impairment, increased risk of falls and accidents (especially in older adults), and a high potential for physical dependence.

Cannabis

With changing laws and social norms, cannabis is a substance you will encounter with increasing frequency. It is important to have a clear understanding of its effects and risks.

- **Common Street Names:** Marijuana, pot, weed, bud. Concentrated forms include hashish, dabs, and wax.

13

- **Mechanism of Action:** The primary psychoactive compound, delta-9-tetrahydrocannabinol (THC), acts on cannabinoid receptors in the brain, which are involved in memory, pleasure, concentration, and time perception.

- **Signs of Intoxication:** Red eyes, increased heart rate, dry mouth, and increased appetite. Psychologically, effects can range from euphoria and relaxation to anxiety and paranoia, especially with high-potency products.

- **Withdrawal Syndrome and Timeline:** Once thought not to exist, cannabis withdrawal is now well-documented, especially in individuals with heavy, daily use. While not life-threatening, it can be very uncomfortable. Symptoms include irritability, anxiety, insomnia, decreased appetite, and restlessness.

- **Long-Term Health Consequences:** Chronic bronchitis (if smoked), potential for impaired cognitive function with long-term heavy use, and the risk of **Cannabinoid Hyperemesis Syndrome**—a condition characterized by cyclical, severe nausea and vomiting in chronic users, often relieved only by hot showers.

Case Examples in Practice

Case Example 1: Sarah, the Overdose in the ED

Sarah, a 22-year-old, is brought in by her friends who say she "used some H and then just went out." On arrival, she is cyanotic, with a respiratory rate of 4 breaths per minute and pinpoint pupils.

- **Clinical Recognition:** The nurse immediately recognizes the opioid triad. Her first thoughts are not about judgment, but about the ABCs—Airway, Breathing, Circulation.

- **Intervention:** While another team member applies oxygen via a bag-valve mask, the nurse establishes IV access. The physician orders 2 mg of naloxone IV push. The nurse administers the medication, and within a minute, Sarah gasps, her eyes fly open, and she sits up, confused and agitated. The nurse knows this abrupt awakening is not a sign of recovery but the beginning of acute withdrawal. She speaks calmly, "Sarah, you're in the hospital. You had an overdose, and we gave you medicine to help you breathe. I know you feel awful right now. We're here to help." The priority shifts from rescue to managing withdrawal and providing a safe, supportive environment.

Case Example 2: Mr. Chen, the Surgical Patient in Withdrawal

Mr. Chen, 62, is on the medical-surgical floor recovering from a colon resection. On post-op day two, his nurse notes he is increasingly anxious, sweaty, and has a noticeable hand tremor. His heart rate is 120 bpm and his blood pressure is 170/98 mmHg. He has been irritable with his family and is complaining of seeing "bugs" on the wall.

- **Clinical Recognition:** The nurse does not dismiss this as post-operative confusion. The constellation of symptoms—autonomic hyperactivity (tachycardia, hypertension, sweating), tremor, and visual hallucinations—screams alcohol withdrawal.

- **Intervention:** She immediately notifies the surgical resident and suggests using a validated tool like the CIWA-Ar (Clinical Institute Withdrawal Assessment for Alcohol, Revised) scale to quantify the severity of the withdrawal. Based on his high score, the team initiates a symptom-triggered protocol with lorazepam. The nurse administers the first dose and continues to monitor Mr. Chen closely, explaining to him and his family what is happening in a calm, factual manner. Her early recognition and intervention prevent his progression to full-blown delirium tremens.

Case Example 3: Jessica, the Agitated College Student

Jessica, 20, is brought to the ED by campus police. She is pacing, yelling, and appears to be responding to internal stimuli. Her pupils are widely dilated, and she is sweating profusely despite the cool temperature of the room. Her heart rate is 140 bpm.

- **Clinical Recognition:** The nurse recognizes the signs of severe stimulant intoxication. The key is to differentiate this from a primary psychotic episode, though clinically, the initial management is similar.

- **Intervention:** The first priority is safety—for Jessica and the staff. The nurse ensures the room is clear of unnecessary equipment, speaks in a low, calm voice, and avoids challenging Jessica's paranoid beliefs. The medical team orders a benzodiazepine to manage her agitation and tachycardia. The nurse's goal is to create a low-stimulus environment to help "talk her down" while the medication takes effect. Once she is calm, the nurse can begin to gather a history and provide education and resources.

A Final Word on Clinical Readiness

This chapter has armed you with the essential, need-to-know information for managing patients who use substances. Your ability to quickly recognize these patterns of intoxication and withdrawal is not just an academic exercise—it is a fundamental nursing skill that saves lives. It allows you to anticipate needs, prevent complications, and intervene with confidence and compassion. You are now equipped with the "what." In the chapters that follow, we will build upon this foundation, moving into the "how"—the skills and strategies you can use to effectively screen, assess, and motivate your patients toward a path of recovery.

Key Takeaways for Your Practice

- Rapidly identify the classic signs of opioid intoxication (pinpoint pupils, respiratory depression) and be prepared to administer naloxone.

- Alcohol and benzodiazepine withdrawal are medical emergencies that can be fatal; maintain a high index of suspicion and advocate for prompt treatment with a validated protocol.

- Stimulant intoxication presents with an over-activated state (tachycardia, hypertension, agitation); prioritize cardiac monitoring and de-escalation.

- Recognize that withdrawal from any substance, even if not life-threatening, causes profound distress and requires a compassionate, supportive nursing response.

Chapter 3: Screening, Brief Intervention, and Referral to Treatment (SBIRT)

The Nurse's Role

You are at the end of a long shift. You have a patient to discharge, another to admit, and three call bells are going off simultaneously. The last thing you feel you have time for is a lengthy conversation about substance use with every patient who comes through the door. This is a real and valid concern. So let's be clear from the outset: this chapter is not about adding an impossibly time-consuming task to your already overflowing plate. It is about introducing a highly efficient, evidence-based tool that allows you to make a profound difference in just a few minutes. That tool is SBIRT. Think of it less as a complex new procedure and more like taking a vital sign—a vital sign for behavioral health.

What Exactly Is SBIRT?

SBIRT is a public health approach for delivering early intervention and treatment services for people with—or at risk of developing—substance use disorders. It is designed for use in general healthcare settings like primary care clinics, hospital emergency departments, and community health centers. The power of SBIRT is that it allows us to identify and help people who may not be seeking treatment for their substance use and whose use might otherwise go unnoticed until it becomes a crisis.

It consists of three straightforward components:

1. **Screening:** Quickly assessing a patient for risky substance use behaviors using standardized tools.

2. **Brief Intervention:** A short, motivational, and awareness-raising conversation with patients whose screening indicates risky use.

3. **Referral to Treatment:** Helping patients who need more extensive treatment to access specialty care.

As a nurse, you are perfectly positioned to deliver SBIRT. You are on the front lines, you are a trusted source of health information, and you are skilled at building rapport with patients quickly. Let's examine how to put this into practice.

The First Step: Universal Screening

The goal of screening is to universally—and quickly—identify individuals who are using substances in a way that could put their health at risk. Just as we screen everyone for high blood pressure, not just those who look unwell, we screen everyone for risky substance use. This normalizes the conversation and removes the stigma of being singled out.

The key to successful screening is to use a validated tool and introduce it as a routine part of care. You might say: **"As part of our commitment to your overall health, we ask all of our patients a few questions about their use of alcohol and other substances. Would you be comfortable answering them?"**

Two of the most common and effective tools are the AUDIT for alcohol and the DAST-10 for other drugs.

The AUDIT (Alcohol Use Disorders Identification Test)

This is a 10-question tool developed by the World Health Organization (WHO) that asks about the quantity of alcohol consumed, symptoms of dependence, and negative consequences of use.

Instructions: Ask the patient the following questions.

1. How often do you have a drink containing alcohol? (0=Never, 1=Monthly or less, 2=2-4 times a month, 3=2-3 times a week, 4=4 or more times a week)

2. How many standard drinks containing alcohol do you have on a typical day when you are drinking? (0=1 or 2, 1=3 or 4, 2=5 or 6, 3=7 to 9, 4=10 or more)

3. How often do you have six or more standard drinks on one occasion? (0=Never, 1=Less than monthly, 2=Monthly, 3=Weekly, 4=Daily or almost daily)

4. How often during the last year have you found that you were not able to stop drinking once you had started? (0=Never, 1=Less than monthly, 2=Monthly, 3=Weekly, 4=Daily or almost daily)

5. How often during the last year have you failed to do what was normally expected from you because of drinking? (0=Never, 1=Less than monthly, 2=Monthly, 3=Weekly, 4=Daily or almost daily)

6. How often during the last year have you needed a first drink in the morning to get yourself going after a heavy drinking session? (0=Never, 1=Less than monthly, 2=Monthly, 3=Weekly, 4=Daily or almost daily)

7. How often during the last year have you had a feeling of guilt or remorse after drinking? (0=Never, 1=Less than monthly, 2=Monthly, 3=Weekly, 4=Daily or almost daily)[1]

8. How often during the last year have you been unable to remember what happened the night[2] before because you had been drinking? (0=Never, 1=Less than monthly, 2=Monthly, 3=Weekly, 4=Daily or almost daily)[3]

9. Have you or someone else been injured as a result of your drinking? (0=No, 2=Yes, but not i[4]n the last year, 4=Yes, during the last year)

10. Has a relative, friend, doctor, or other health worker been concerned about your drinking or suggested you cut down? (0=No, 2=Yes, but not in the last year, 4=Yes, during the last year)

Scoring the AUDIT:

Add up the points for each answer. The score helps you determine the risk zone.

- **Zone I (0-7 for men, 0-7 for women):** Low Risk. Offer praise and reinforcement.

- **Zone II (8-15):** Risky Use. This is the prime target for a Brief Intervention.

- **Zone III (16-19):** Harmful Use. A Brief Intervention is needed, and a referral should be strongly considered.

- **Zone IV (20-40):** High Risk / Likely Dependence. A Brief Intervention and a direct referral to treatment are necessary.

The DAST-10 (Drug Abuse Screening Test)

This is a 10-question yes/no tool to screen for problematic use of drugs other than alcohol.

Instructions: Ask the patient if they have used drugs other than those required for medical reasons in the past 12 months. If yes, ask the following questions. A "Yes" answer scores 1 point.

1. Have you used drugs other than those required for medical reasons?

2. Do you abuse more than one drug at a time?

3. Are you always able to stop using drugs when you want to? (A "No" answer counts as a "Yes" for scoring)

4. Have you ever had blackouts or flashbacks as a result of drug use?[5]

5. Do you ever feel bad or guilty about your drug use?[6]

6. Does your spouse (or parents) ever complain about your involvement with drugs?[7]

7. Have you neglected your family because of your use of drugs?[8]

8. Have you engaged in illegal activ⁹ities to obtain drugs?

9. Have you ever experienced withdrawal symptoms (felt sick) when you stopped taking drugs?

10. Have you had medical problems as a result of your drug use (e.g., memory loss, hepatitis, convulsions, bleeding)?

Scoring the DAST-10:

Add up the points.

- **0:** No problem reported.

- **1-2:** Low Risk. Provide feedback and monitor.

- **3-5:** Moderate Risk / Harmful Use. Brief Intervention is needed.

- **6-10:** High Risk / Severe Use. Brief Intervention and referral to treatment are necessary.

The Second Step: Brief Intervention

So, your patient's score falls into Zone II on the AUDIT. Now what? This is where the Brief Intervention (BI) comes in. This is not a lecture. It is not a confrontation. It is a 5-to-10-minute collaborative conversation that uses motivational principles to raise the patient's awareness and encourage them to think about making a change.

Here is a simple framework for conducting a BI:

1. **Ask Permission & Share the Results:** "Would it be okay if we spent a few minutes talking about your screening results?"

2. **Provide Feedback:** "Your score was a 12 on the alcohol screen. This score falls into a range that we consider risky for your health. I'd like to share some information about that if you're open to it."

3. **Link to Their Health:** Connect their substance use to their presenting complaint or their health goals. "You mentioned

you want to get your blood pressure down. Drinking at this level can make that harder to achieve."

4. **Elicit Their Reaction:** Ask them what they think. "What are your thoughts on that?" or "How does that information fit with how you see your own drinking?"

5. **Discuss Low-Risk Guidelines:** Provide clear, non-judgmental information. "For men, low-risk drinking is considered no more than four drinks on any single day and no more than 14 drinks per week. For women, it's no more than three on any day and seven per week. Your use is a bit above those levels."

6. **Explore Readiness and Set a Goal:** Ask them where they stand. "On a scale from 0 to 10, where 0 is not at all ready and 10 is completely ready, how ready are you to think about making a change in your drinking?" Whatever their answer, your goal is to help them identify a small, achievable next step.

The Third Step: Referral to Treatment

For patients with a high screening score or clear signs of a severe substance use disorder, a BI alone is not enough. They need a **Referral to Treatment (RT)**. But simply handing someone a phone number is rarely effective. The most effective method is a **"warm handoff."**

A warm handoff means making a direct, active connection between the patient and the treatment provider. It transforms the referral from an abstract idea into a concrete action.

- **In a hospital setting,** this could mean calling the social worker or a substance use liaison nurse to come and meet the patient at the bedside before they are discharged.

- **In a clinic setting,** it could mean walking the patient down the hall to the behavioral health provider's office and making a personal introduction: "Maria, this is John. He's one of our counselors. I've told him a little bit about what you're looking for, and he's ready to help you schedule an appointment."

The key is to facilitate a direct connection, which dramatically increases the likelihood that the patient will follow through.

Case Examples in Practice

Case Example 1: Mark in the Emergency Department

Mark, a 45-year-old construction worker, comes to the ED after falling from a ladder and fracturing his ankle. As part of the intake, the triage nurse administers the AUDIT. Mark scores a 16.

- **Screening:** The nurse flags the score.

- **Brief Intervention:** After Mark's ankle has been stabilized, the nurse finds a quiet moment. "Mark, I see from the health screen you filled out that your score for alcohol use was a 16. That's a level where we sometimes see health problems develop. Would you be open to talking about that for a minute?" Mark shrugs. The nurse continues, "Sometimes when people drink at this level, it can affect their balance and coordination. I wonder if that might have played a role in your fall today?" Mark looks down and nods. "Maybe." The nurse provides the low-risk guidelines and asks, "What do you think about that?" This brief conversation plants a seed, linking his drinking directly to a negative consequence. She provides him with a handout and says, "Maybe this is something to think about while your ankle is healing."

Case Example 2: The "Joan" Scenario in an OB-GYN Clinic

Joan, 25, is 10 weeks pregnant and comes for her first prenatal visit. She completes the screening forms, scoring a 9 on the AUDIT. The

24

nurse knows that *any* alcohol use during pregnancy is risky. (This scenario is adapted from the University of Pittsburgh's excellent SBIRT training [2]).

- **Nurse:** "Joan, thanks for filling out these forms. I see on the health questionnaire you answered that you have a few drinks a week. Can you tell me more about that?"

- **Joan:** "Oh, it's nothing really. Just a glass or two of wine at night to relax."

- **Nurse (empathetic, non-judgmental):** "A lot of women find that helps them unwind. And since you're now pregnant, this is a good time to talk about what's safest for the baby. We now know that no amount of alcohol has been proven safe during pregnancy. What are your thoughts about that?"

- **Joan (worried):** "Oh, I didn't know that. I definitely don't want to hurt my baby."

- **Nurse (offering a plan):** "That's great, Joan. That tells me you're already thinking about how to have the healthiest pregnancy possible. How about we set a goal of stopping alcohol completely for the rest of your pregnancy? I can also connect you with some resources that offer great support for new moms."

This non-confrontational, educational approach empowers Joan to make a healthy choice without shaming her.

Case Example 3: Frank in Primary Care

Frank, 68, a retired accountant, comes in for his annual physical. His blood pressure is elevated, and his lab work shows slightly elevated liver enzymes. He completes the DAST-10 and scores a 4, noting that he uses his wife's leftover oxycodone from a past surgery "to help with my arthritis."

- **Screening:** The nurse sees the elevated DAST score combined with the concerning clinical signs.

- **Brief Intervention & Referral:** "Frank, thanks for being so honest on this form. I see you noted using oxycodone for your arthritis, and you scored a 4 on the screening. That score, combined with the changes in your bloodwork, suggests that this medication might be causing some harm. What are your thoughts about that?" Frank admits he's been taking more than he should and feels "a little lost without it."

- **Warm Handoff:** The nurse recognizes this goes beyond a simple BI. She says, "It sounds like this has become more than you can manage on your own, and that's okay. We have a behavioral health specialist, Sarah, right here in our clinic. She's an expert in helping people find safer ways to manage pain. Would you be willing to chat with her for a few minutes today? I can introduce you." The nurse walks Frank down the hall and personally introduces him to Sarah, who schedules an intake appointment. This warm handoff makes it much more likely that Frank will engage in treatment.

A Final Thought on Seizing the Moment

As nurses, we are granted brief, fleeting moments of connection with our patients. SBIRT is a framework that allows us to make the most of those moments. It is a structured, efficient way to turn a routine check-up into a potential turning point. It is not about becoming an addiction specialist overnight. It is about recognizing risk, opening a conversation, and knowing when and how to connect a person with the help they need. It is about planting a seed of change that can, with the right care, grow into a life saved.

Key Takeaways for Your Practice

- Implement universal screening for substance use as a standard of care, just like checking blood pressure.

- A Brief Intervention is a collaborative conversation, not a lecture. Your goal is to raise awareness and let the patient be the expert on their own life.

- Link a patient's substance use directly to their health goals or their reason for seeking care.

- When a patient needs more help, a "warm handoff" to a specialist is far more effective than just providing a phone number.

Having learned how to identify risk and open the door to conversation with SBIRT, we now need to perfect the art of that conversation itself. We need to learn the language of change. That is the work of Motivational Interviewing.

Chapter 4: Motivational Interviewing (MI)

The Language of Change

If SBIRT is the tool that opens the door, then Motivational Interviewing (MI) is the skill that allows you to walk through it with your patient. It is the language we use to help people find their own reasons for making a change. You might be thinking that "motivating people" sounds like being a cheerleader, or worse, like trying to argue someone into a different way of living. It is neither. In fact, if you find yourself arguing with a patient, you are no longer doing MI. Motivational Interviewing, at its core, is a profound act of listening. It is a way of being with a person that honors their autonomy and helps them untangle their own ambivalence about change. As nurses, much of this will feel deeply familiar—it aligns perfectly with our professional ethos of patient-centered care.

The Spirit of Motivational Interviewing

Before we get into the techniques and strategies, we must first understand the "spirit" of MI. Without this underlying mindset, the techniques will feel hollow and manipulative. This spirit was defined by the founders of MI, William Miller and Stephen Rollnick, and it consists of four interconnected elements [3].

1. **Partnership:** You are not the expert wrestling with a passive patient. You are in a collaborative partnership, working alongside your patient. They are the expert on their life, their values, and their challenges. You bring clinical expertise, but the work is done together.

2. **Acceptance:** This involves four aspects:

   - **Absolute Worth:** You value the patient as a fellow human being, without judgment.

   - **Accurate Empathy:** You make an active effort to understand the patient's world from their perspective.

o   **Autonomy Support:** You honor their right and capacity to make their own decisions—including the decision not to change.

o   **Affirmation:** You actively seek out and acknowledge the patient's strengths and efforts.

3. **Compassion:** This is more than just feeling for someone. It is an active commitment to promote the other's welfare, to have their best interests at heart.

4. **Evocation:** This is perhaps the most unique element. The belief here is that the motivation for change does not come from you; it is already inside the patient. Your job is not to install it but to *evoke* it—to draw it out. You are helping them find their *own* reasons.

The Four Processes of MI

A conversation in MI has a natural flow. Think of it as a journey you take with the patient, guided by four processes.

1. **Engaging:** This is the foundation. Your first task is to build rapport and establish a trusting working relationship. If the patient does not feel comfortable and respected, nothing else can happen.

2. **Focusing:** Once engaged, you and the patient collaboratively decide on a direction. Out of all the things you *could* talk about, what will you talk about? It's about developing a specific target for change.

3. **Evoking:** This is the heart of MI. Having agreed on a focus, you now elicit the patient's own motivations for change. You are listening for and encouraging "change talk"—the patient's own arguments for change.

4. **Planning:** When the patient's change talk becomes strong and consistent, you can move to planning. This involves

developing a concrete, acceptable, and achievable plan of action.

The Core Skills: Your MI Toolkit (OARS)

The spirit and processes of MI are put into action through a set of core communication skills, neatly summarized by the acronym **OARS**.

- **O**pen Questions
- **A**ffirmations
- **R**eflections
- **S**ummaries

Let's look at each of these in detail.

Open Questions

An open question is one that cannot be answered with a simple "yes" or "no." It invites the patient to think, explore, and elaborate. It opens the door to conversation.

- **Instead of:** "Do you want to quit smoking?" (Closed)
- **Try:** "What are some of the things you don't like about smoking?" (Open)
- **Instead of:** "Are you taking your medication?" (Closed)
- **Try:** "How has it been going with your new medication plan?" (Open)

Affirmations

An affirmation is a direct statement of recognition for a patient's strengths, efforts, or positive qualities. It is not praise; it is a genuine acknowledgment. Affirmations build confidence and self-efficacy. They tell the patient, "I see you, and I see the good in you."

- "You've been through a lot, and you're still here, still trying. That shows a lot of resilience."

- "That was a really honest thing to say. I appreciate you sharing that with me."

- "You're a good parent. It's clear how much you care about your kids."

Reflections

Reflections are the most important skill in MI. A reflection is a statement, not a question, that reflects back the meaning of what the patient has just said. It shows you are listening and allows the patient to hear their own thoughts, feelings, and motivations played back to them.

- **Simple Reflection:** Repeats or slightly rephrases what the patient said.

  - **Patient:** "I'm just so tired of being sick all the time."

  - **Nurse:** "You're feeling worn out by it all."

- **Complex Reflection:** Makes a guess about the underlying meaning or feeling. This is where the magic happens.

  - **Patient:** "My wife is always nagging me about my drinking. I wish she would just get off my back."

  - **Nurse:** "It feels like no matter what you do, you can't please her, and it's frustrating." (Reflecting the feeling of frustration and being misunderstood, rather than the "nagging").

  - Patient: "Exactly! And I mean, I know she's right, but..."

That "but" is the opening you are looking for.

Summaries

A summary is essentially a collection of reflections. It pulls together the key points of the conversation, allowing you and the patient to see the whole picture. A good summary often highlights the patient's ambivalence—the push and pull of their feelings—and can be used to transition to the next step.

- "So, let me see if I have this right. On the one hand, drinking wine at night is one of the only ways you've found to relax and get a break from the stress of your job. On the other hand, you're worried about what it's doing to your health, you're tired of feeling groggy in the morning, and you're concerned about the example it sets for your kids. Did I get that about right?"

This kind of summary sets the stage for a key question: **"Where does this leave you now?"**

Case Examples in Practice

Case Example 1: David, the Diabetic Patient

David, 52, has type 2 diabetes. His A1c is high, and he confides in the clinic nurse that he rarely checks his blood sugar.

- **The Wrong Way (Confrontational):** "David, you have to check your sugars. If you don't, you could lose a foot or go blind. Do you understand?" (This elicits defensiveness).

- **The MI Way (Engaging & Evoking):**

  - **Nurse (Open Question):** "David, help me understand. What makes it difficult to check your blood sugar regularly?"

  - **David:** "I don't know... I hate seeing high numbers. It just makes me feel like a failure."

  - **Nurse (Complex Reflection):** "So the number on the screen feels like a judgment, and it's just easier not to look than to face that feeling."

  - **David:** "Yeah, that's it exactly."

- ○ **Nurse (Affirmation):** "Thank you for saying that. It takes courage to be that honest, and it helps me understand."

- ○ **Nurse (Evoking Change Talk):** "What do you think might be one good thing about getting into the habit of checking it more often?"

- ○ **David:** "Well, I guess I'd know where I stand. And my wife would stop worrying so much."

- ○ **Nurse:** "So it would give you a sense of control and maybe bring some peace of mind at home." (Reflecting the change talk).

Case Example 2: Brenda, the ER Patient

Brenda, 34, is in the ER for the third time in a year with injuries from a domestic partner. While patching up a cut on her arm, the nurse wants to open a conversation.

- **Nurse (Engaging with Empathy):** "This looks really painful. And this isn't the first time you've been hurt like this."

- **Brenda:** "I'm fine. I just... I fell."

- **Nurse (Acceptance & Reflection):** "It's difficult and scary to talk about these things. And you're trying to protect yourself." (Instead of challenging the lie, the nurse reflects the underlying feeling).

- **Brenda (starts to cry):** "He promised he would stop."

- **Nurse (Affirmation):** "You believed in him, and you wanted the relationship to work. You've been trying so hard to hold everything together."

- **Nurse (Open Question):** "On a scale from 1 to 10, how safe do you feel going home today?"

- **Brenda:** "Maybe a 3."

- **Nurse (Evoking):** "What would it take to get that number to a 4 or a 5? What's one small thing that might make you feel even a little bit safer?"

This approach doesn't force a solution. It honors Brenda's fear and ambivalence while gently exploring possibilities and building a safety plan, one step at a time. Michelle Dart's work on MI in nursing practice highlights how these brief, empathetic interactions can be incredibly powerful [4].

Case Example 3: Michael, Considering Medication-Assisted Treatment

Michael, 28, has an opioid use disorder and is ambivalent about starting buprenorphine.

- **Michael:** "I don't know. I feel like taking buprenorphine is just trading one drug for another. Isn't it just a crutch?"

- **Nurse (Complex Reflection):** "So you're worried about becoming dependent on something else, and you value the idea of being completely free from any substance."

- **Michael:** "Right! I want to be *clean*."

- **Nurse (Providing Information with Permission):** "I hear that. The desire to be completely substance-free is a powerful goal. Would it be okay if I shared how some other patients have thought about it?" (Waits for a nod). "Some people see it less as a crutch and more like insulin for a person with diabetes. It's a medication that treats the underlying brain changes, quiets the cravings—that 'hungry ghost' we talked about— and gives them the stability to work on all the other parts of their recovery. What are your thoughts on that way of looking at it?"

- **Michael:** "I never thought of it like that. So it would stop the cravings?"

- **Nurse (Summarizing):** "It sounds like on one side, you have this important value of being completely drug-free. And on the other, the idea of finally getting some relief from the constant cravings is appealing. That's a tough spot to be in." This summary validates his conflict without taking a side, allowing him to be the one to resolve his own ambivalence.

Final Reflections on the Language of Care

Motivational Interviewing is not a trick to get patients to do what we want. It is a fundamental shift in the way we communicate. It is a disciplined and humble practice of setting aside our own agenda to truly listen to the person in front of us. It is the belief that our patients possess the wisdom and motivation to heal, and that our role is to help them discover it. It is, in short, the language of hope, and it is a language every nurse can, and should, learn to speak fluently.

Key Takeaways for Your Practice

- Adopt the "spirit" of MI: Be a partner, not a director. Offer acceptance, compassion, and evoke the patient's own wisdom.

- Master the OARS: Use **O**pen questions to invite conversation, **A**ffirmations to build confidence, **R**eflections to show you're listening, and **S**ummaries to tie it all together.

- Listen for "change talk"—any statement the patient makes in favor of change—and reflect it back. This is the fuel for the engine of change.

- Resist the "righting reflex"—the natural urge to fix problems and give advice. Let the patient be the agent of their own change.

Chapter 5: Managing Withdrawal

The Nursing Care Plan

There are few clinical situations as raw or as challenging as caring for a person in acute withdrawal. It is a physiological and psychological storm, and you, the nurse, are the lighthouse. Your patient may be trembling, sweating, seeing things that are not there, or curled in a ball of misery, every muscle aching. In these moments, it is easy to feel overwhelmed. But this is where the structure and discipline of the nursing process become your most powerful allies. This is not a time for guesswork. It is a time for systematic assessment, precise intervention, and unwavering compassion. This chapter will provide you with the framework to navigate that storm safely and effectively.

Assessment: Your Eyes, Ears, and Scales

Your primary responsibility in managing withdrawal is vigilant assessment. You are the frontline observer, the one who will detect subtle changes before they become catastrophic emergencies. While your clinical judgment is indispensable, it must be paired with the use of objective, validated scales. These tools do two things: they provide a common language for the entire healthcare team, and they help you quantify the severity of withdrawal, which in turn guides treatment—especially symptom-triggered therapy.

The CIWA-Ar (Clinical Institute Withdrawal Assessment for Alcohol, Revised)

For alcohol withdrawal—and often for benzodiazepine withdrawal as well—the CIWA-Ar is the gold standard. It is a 10-item scale that assesses symptoms like nausea, tremor, anxiety, agitation, and disorientation. Each item is scored, and the total score dictates the level of intervention required.

- **How to Use It:** You will sit with the patient and ask a series of questions ("Do you feel sick to your stomach?" "Do you feel nervous?") while also observing them for signs like tremor and sweating. You then score each category. For example, tremor is scored from 0 (no tremor) to 7 (severe, continuous tremor).

- **What the Score Means:** A score below 8 or 10 typically requires only supportive care. Scores in the 10-18 range indicate moderate withdrawal and usually warrant medication. A score of 19 or higher signifies severe withdrawal and a high risk of seizures or delirium tremens, requiring immediate and aggressive treatment. The beauty of a symptom-triggered protocol is that you treat what you see, providing medication when the patient needs it and holding it when they do not.

The COWS (Clinical Opiate Withdrawal Scale)

For opioid withdrawal, the COWS is your tool of choice. It is an 11-item scale that measures objective signs like resting pulse rate, pupil size, and piloerection (goosebumps), as well as patient-reported symptoms like bone aches and anxiety.

- **How to Use It:** You will take vital signs and observe the patient, then ask them to rate their experience. The scores are tallied to determine the level of withdrawal.

- **What the Score Means:** A score of 5-12 indicates mild withdrawal. 13-24 is moderate, 25-36 is moderately severe, and a score over 36 is severe withdrawal. The COWS is critically important not just for providing comfort, but also for determining the right time to start Medication-Assisted Treatment like buprenorphine, which we will discuss in the next chapter.

The Nursing Care Plan: A Framework for Action

Let's structure our approach using the nursing care plan format you know well. We will focus on the most common and dangerous withdrawal syndromes.

Nursing Care Plan: Alcohol Withdrawal

Patient Profile: A 58-year-old man admitted to the hospital for pneumonia who has a history of drinking a pint of vodka daily. It is now 36 hours since his last drink. His CIWA-Ar score is 22.

- **Nursing Diagnosis 1: Risk for Injury** related to central nervous system stimulation (seizures, delirium) as evidenced by a high CIWA-Ar score, confusion, and agitation.

    - **Goal:** The patient will remain free from injury throughout the withdrawal period.

    - **Interventions:**

        1. **Implement seizure precautions:** Pad the side rails, ensure suction equipment is at the bedside. **Rationale:** To prevent injury in the event of a tonic-clonic seizure, a known complication of severe alcohol withdrawal.

        2. **Administer benzodiazepines (e.g., lorazepam, diazepam) as prescribed based on the CIWA-Ar protocol. Rationale:** Benzodiazepines are the first-line treatment. They work on the same GABA receptors as alcohol, effectively acting as a substitute to calm the overexcited central nervous system and prevent progression to seizures and delirium.

        3. **Maintain a low-stimulus environment:** Dim the lights, reduce noise, limit visitors. **Rationale:** An overexcited brain is highly sensitive to external stimuli, which can worsen agitation and confusion.

        4. **Reorient the patient frequently:** State your name, the place, and the date. Use a calm, clear voice. **Rationale:** To decrease the fear and confusion associated with delirium.

- **Nursing Diagnosis 2: Risk for Deficient Fluid Volume** related to diaphoresis, vomiting, and decreased oral intake.

  - **Goal:** The patient will maintain adequate hydration, as evidenced by moist mucous membranes and good urine output.

  - **Interventions:**

    1. **Monitor intake and output closely. Rationale:** To provide an objective measure of fluid balance.

    2. **Encourage oral fluids as tolerated.** Offer water, broth, or electrolyte-containing drinks. **Rationale:** To replace fluid and electrolytes lost through sweating and vomiting.

    3. **Administer intravenous fluids as ordered. Rationale:** To ensure adequate hydration when the patient is unable to tolerate oral intake.

Nursing Care Plan: Opioid Withdrawal

Patient Profile: A 24-year-old woman presenting to the emergency department requesting help. Her last use of heroin was 14 hours ago. Her COWS score is 18.

- **Nursing Diagnosis 1: Acute Pain** related to physiological effects of opioid withdrawal as evidenced by patient reports of diffuse muscle and bone aches and a COWS score of 18.

  - **Goal:** The patient will report a decrease in pain to a manageable level.

  - **Interventions:**

    1. **Administer non-opioid comfort medications as prescribed.** This may include clonidine for autonomic symptoms (like anxiety and tachycardia) and NSAIDs (like ibuprofen) for

muscle aches. **Rationale:** To provide symptomatic relief without using opioids.

2. **Provide non-pharmacological comfort measures:** Offer warm blankets or a hot shower, gentle repositioning, and distraction techniques. **Rationale:** These measures can help soothe aching muscles and provide psychological comfort.

- **Nursing Diagnosis 2: Ineffective Coping** related to intense cravings and psychological distress as evidenced by statements like, "I can't take this, I need to use."

  o **Goal:** The patient will identify at least one positive coping strategy.

  o **Interventions:**

    1. **Provide continuous emotional support and reassurance.** Stay with the patient as much as possible. Say, "I know this is incredibly difficult, but it will not last forever. I am here with you." **Rationale:** The presence of a calm, supportive person can decrease anxiety and help the patient feel less alone in their misery.

    2. **Acknowledge the reality of their discomfort without judgment.** Validate their experience. "It makes sense that you feel this way. This is a very tough process." **Rationale:** Validation builds trust and reduces the shame that can be a barrier to seeking help.

    3. **Reinforce their decision to seek help.** "The fact that you are here, going through this, shows incredible strength and a desire for a different life." **Rationale:** This is an affirmation that builds self-efficacy and reinforces their motivation for change.

Case Examples in Practice

Case Example 1: George on the Med-Surg Floor

George, 65, is admitted for a COPD exacerbation. He is a "social drinker," according to his chart. On his second hospital day, you notice he has a fine tremor in his hands, is sweating despite the room being cool, and seems increasingly anxious. You suspect alcohol withdrawal. You grab a CIWA-Ar form and assess him. His score is 14. You immediately contact the hospitalist, report your findings using the specific language of the scale, and suggest initiating the hospital's symptom-triggered withdrawal protocol. The provider agrees, and you administer the first dose of lorazepam. By performing a proactive assessment with a validated tool, you have prevented George's withdrawal from escalating into a life-threatening emergency.

Case Example 2: Chloe in the Clinic

Chloe, 29, comes to the outpatient addiction clinic for her first appointment. She wants to start on buprenorphine for her fentanyl use disorder. For the induction to be safe, she must be in moderate withdrawal. If she takes the buprenorphine too soon, it will cause precipitated withdrawal—a sudden and severe worsening of symptoms. Your job is to assess her using the COWS scale. You take her pulse (110 bpm), check her pupils (dilated), and note her restlessness and complaints of bone aches. Her final COWS score is 15. You report this to the nurse practitioner, who agrees she is ready. You have used the scale not just for comfort, but as a critical safety check to ensure the successful start of a life-saving medication.

Case Example 3: Mrs. Diaz and Her Valium

Mrs. Diaz, a 72-year-old widow, is brought to the hospital after a fall. The team learns she has been taking diazepam prescribed by a doctor years ago for "nerves," and has been increasing the dose on her own. The decision is made to slowly taper her off the medication. Your role is not just to administer the decreasing doses of the medication, but to manage her profound anxiety. You create a care

41

plan focused on *Ineffective Coping*. Your interventions include teaching her deep breathing exercises, ensuring a sleep-aid tea is available for her at night, and spending time with her, simply listening to her fears about living without the medication that has been her companion for so long. Your non-pharmacological support is just as important as the medication taper in helping her succeed.

Chapter 6: Medication-Assisted Treatment (MAT)

A Nurse's Guide to Buprenorphine, Naltrexone, and Methadone

Let's clear the air on this topic right away. You will hear people—sometimes even other healthcare professionals—say that Medication-Assisted Treatment is "just trading one drug for another." This statement is not only incorrect, it is dangerous. It perpetuates stigma and creates barriers to the single most effective treatment we have for opioid use disorder. So, let's reframe this. We do not call insulin for diabetes "trading one sugar for another." We do not call an inhaler for asthma "trading one breathing problem for another." These are medications that treat chronic medical conditions. MAT is no different. It is the use of medications, in combination with counseling and behavioral therapies, to provide a whole-person approach to the treatment of substance use disorders. As a nurse, you are a key player in dispelling the myths and supporting patients on this life-saving path.

Demystifying the Medications

To be an effective educator and advocate, you need a solid, straightforward understanding of the three main medications used for opioid use disorder (MOUD).

Buprenorphine

- **How it Works:** Buprenorphine is a **partial opioid agonist**. Think of it this way: the opioid receptors in the brain are like locks. A full agonist like heroin or fentanyl is a key that fits the lock perfectly and turns it all the way, producing a powerful high. Buprenorphine is a key that also fits the lock, but it only turns it partway. This is enough to stop withdrawal and reduce cravings, but it does not produce the same intense euphoria. It also has a "ceiling effect," meaning that after a certain dose, taking more does not produce a greater effect, which significantly increases its safety profile compared to full agonists. It is often combined with naloxone (in a product called Suboxone) to deter misuse.

- **The Nurse's Role:** Your role is central, especially during the **induction** phase. You will use the COWS scale to ensure the patient is in adequate withdrawal before the first dose, administer the medication (often as a sublingual film), and then monitor the patient closely for improvement in their symptoms and for any side effects. In the maintenance phase, you provide ongoing education, manage side effects like constipation, and may administer long-acting injectable forms of buprenorphine.

Naltrexone

- **How it Works:** Naltrexone is an **opioid antagonist**. It is a key that fits the lock but completely blocks it, preventing any other opioid key from getting in and working. It does not relieve cravings in the same way buprenorphine does, but it completely removes the rewarding effect of using opioids. A person taking naltrexone who then uses heroin will feel nothing, which can help to extinguish the learned behavior. It is available as a daily pill or a monthly long-acting injection.

- **The Nurse's Role:** Education is paramount. The patient *must* be completely opioid-free for 7-10 days before starting naltrexone to avoid causing sudden, severe withdrawal. Your role is to confirm this, educate the patient on the risks, and administer the long-acting injection. You will also provide support and counseling, as the patient will not have the same "safety net" for cravings that buprenorphine provides.

Methadone

- **How it Works:** Methadone is a **long-acting full opioid agonist**. It is a key that fits the lock and turns it all the way, but it does so very slowly and steadily. It relieves withdrawal and cravings without causing the chaotic cycle of high and crash associated with short-acting opioids like heroin. Because it is a full agonist with no ceiling effect, it carries a higher risk of overdose and is therefore dispensed only through highly regulated Opioid Treatment Programs (OTPs), often called methadone clinics.

- **The Nurse's Role:** Nurses in OTPs are responsible for dispensing the daily dose of methadone, assessing patients for sedation or other side effects, and providing ongoing health education and counseling. For nurses outside of OTPs, the role is one of care coordination—knowing that your patient is on methadone, understanding the importance of their daily dose, and educating them about dangerous drug interactions, especially with benzodiazepines.

Your Role in Action: Patient Education and Support

Regardless of the specific medication, your core role is one of patient education and unwavering support.

- **Explaining the "Why":** You must be able to explain the rationale for MAT in clear, non-judgmental terms. "This medication works by healing the parts of your brain that have been affected by long-term opioid use. It will help to quiet the cravings and stop the withdrawal symptoms, which will give you the chance to focus on your recovery."

- **Managing Side Effects:** Be proactive. For buprenorphine and methadone, constipation is a near-universal side effect. Do not wait for the patient to complain. Initiate a bowel regimen from day one. Discuss other potential side effects like sweating or sedation and offer practical solutions.

- **Reinforcing Adherence:** Frame medication adherence not as a rule, but as a key part of their recovery plan. "Taking this medication every day is one of the most important things you can do to protect your recovery and stay safe."

- **Observing and Advocating:** You are the one who sees the patient most frequently. You will notice if they seem overly sedated or if they are still struggling with cravings. Your observations and reports to the prescribing provider are essential for proper dose titration and treatment planning.

Case Examples in Practice

Case Example 1: Assisting with a Buprenorphine Induction

You are a nurse in an outpatient clinic. Your patient, Maria, is ready to start buprenorphine. You spend the morning with her, assessing her COWS score every hour. When her score hits 14, you notify the provider. You are instructed to give the first 4mg test dose. You sit with Maria, explain what you are doing, and place the film under her tongue. Over the next hour, you stay with her. You see the restlessness fade, the yawning stop, and the color return to her face. She looks at you and says, "The noise... it's finally quiet." In that moment, you are not just a nurse giving a medication; you are a witness to the beginning of a new life.

Case Example 2: Pre-Release Education for Naltrexone

You work in a county jail. A young man, Kevin, is being released in a week and has opted to receive an injection of long-acting naltrexone. You sit with him for a pre-release counseling session. You explain in very clear terms, "Kevin, this injection will block the effects of any opioids. If you use heroin when you get out, you will not get high, but you will still be at a very high risk of overdose if you try to use enough to override the block. This shot is a tool, a shield, but the real work of recovery still has to be done." You connect him with a peer support specialist he can call the day he gets out. Your education is a critical part of his relapse prevention plan.

Case Example 3: Coordinating Care for a Patient on Methadone

Your patient in the primary care clinic, Mr. Jones, receives a daily dose of methadone from a local OTP. He comes to you for management of his hypertension and diabetes. You know that he was recently prescribed diazepam by a dentist. You immediately recognize the danger. You explain to Mr. Jones, "Mr. Jones, the combination of methadone and diazepam can be very dangerous and can stop your breathing. It is very important that we talk to the dentist and your methadone clinic about this." You facilitate a call between all parties to find a safer alternative for his dental anxiety. Your role as a care coordinator and safety monitor has potentially saved his life.

Chapter 7: Addressing Co-Occurring Disorders

The Dual Diagnosis Challenge

If you have been a nurse for more than about a week, you have cared for a patient with a co-occurring disorder. You just may not have called it that. It was the patient with alcohol use disorder who was also being treated for depression. It was the young person who used cannabis to quiet their anxiety. It was the patient with a stimulant use disorder who presented with paranoia so intense it was indistinguishable from schizophrenia. The reality of our work is this: co-occurring substance use and mental health disorders are the expectation, not the exception. The two are often so deeply intertwined that trying to treat one without addressing the other is like trying to build a house on a foundation of sand. It is doomed to fail. As a nurse, with your holistic view of the patient, you are uniquely suited to be the great integrator of care for these individuals.

The Chicken and the Egg—And Why It Doesn't Matter

Clinicians and researchers can spend a great deal of time debating which came first—the mental illness or the substance use. Did the person start drinking because they were depressed, or did they become depressed because of their long-term alcohol use? From a practical nursing perspective, the answer is often: **yes**. The relationship is bidirectional and synergistic.

- **Self-Medication:** A person with untreated anxiety, trauma, or depression may use substances to temporarily relieve their psychic pain. Alcohol quiets the anxious mind. Opioids numb the emotional agony of PTSD. Stimulants can provide a fleeting antidote to the fatigue and anhedonia of depression.

- **Substance-Induced Disorders:** Conversely, chronic substance use can create or worsen mental illness. Long-term alcohol use is a direct depressant. Stimulant use can cause profound anxiety, paranoia, and psychosis. Withdrawal from nearly any substance can mimic the symptoms of a major anxiety disorder.

The key takeaway for you as a nurse is that you must always assess for both. When you see one, you must look for the other.

The Nurse's Role: An Integrated Approach

The old model of care was sequential: "Go get your drinking under control, and *then* we'll treat your depression." We now know this approach is deeply flawed. A person cannot effectively engage in therapy for their depression if their brain is clouded by daily alcohol use. Likewise, they will find it nearly impossible to stop drinking if the underlying depression driving the use is left untreated. We must move to an **integrated treatment model**, where both conditions are addressed at the same time, by the same team, in the same place. Your role is to champion and facilitate this integration.

Integrated Assessment

Your assessment must be holistic. When you are screening for substance use with the AUDIT or DAST, you should also be screening for common mental health conditions. Simple, validated tools can be easily incorporated into your workflow.

- **For Depression:** The **PHQ-9 (Patient Health Questionnaire-9)** is a quick, 9-question tool that aligns with the diagnostic criteria for major depression.

- **For Anxiety:** The **GAD-7 (Generalized Anxiety Disorder-7)** is a 7-question scale to screen for anxiety.

- **For Trauma:** Simply asking, "Have you ever experienced a traumatic event that still affects you today?" can open the door.

Advocating for Integrated Plans

When you identify a co-occurring disorder, you become an advocate. This means ensuring the treatment plan reflects the patient's full reality. Does the patient being admitted for alcohol withdrawal also have a plan for a psychiatric evaluation? Does the patient starting on MAT for opioid use also have a referral for trauma-informed therapy? You are the one who asks these questions in team meetings and care conferences, ensuring the patient does not fall through the cracks between the mental health system and the substance use treatment system.

Care Coordination

You are the communication hub. You are the one who can talk to the psychiatrist about the patient's progress in their substance use group. You are the one who can talk to the substance use counselor about the new antidepressant the patient was just started on. This communication is essential. For example, some antidepressants can have side effects that might be misinterpreted as withdrawal or intoxication. Without clear communication, treatment plans can work at cross-purposes.

Case Examples in Practice

Case Example 1: Maria, Depression and Alcohol

Maria, 42, is admitted to the medical floor for pancreatitis secondary to alcohol use. You are managing her alcohol withdrawal with a CIWA-Ar protocol. During your conversations, you notice she speaks with a flat affect and expresses feelings of hopelessness. You decide to administer the PHQ-9, and she scores a 21, indicating severe depression. In the discharge planning meeting, the focus is on a referral to an alcohol treatment program. You speak up. "I'm concerned about Maria's depression. Her PHQ-9 was 21. I think it's unlikely she'll be successful in an alcohol program if her severe depression isn't addressed at the same time. Can we get an inpatient psychiatric consult before she leaves to discuss an integrated plan, perhaps including an antidepressant?" Your advocacy directly leads to a more effective, integrated discharge plan.

Case Example 2: Jason, Methamphetamine and Psychosis

Jason, a 22-year-old, is brought to the ED by police for bizarre and agitated behavior. He is paranoid, responding to internal stimuli, and has not slept in three days. His urine drug screen is positive for amphetamines. The immediate priority is ensuring his safety and the safety of the staff. You work to create a calm, non-threatening environment, speaking in a low, clear voice. The medical team treats his agitation with a benzodiazepine. The question arises: is this a primary psychotic disorder like schizophrenia, or is it substance-induced? Your role is not to make that diagnosis, but to treat the presenting symptoms and communicate your observations clearly to both the medical and psychiatric teams. You document his vital signs, his response to medication, and the content of his paranoid thoughts. Your detailed notes will be essential for the psychiatric consultant to make an accurate diagnosis and treatment plan once the acute intoxication has resolved.

Case Example 3: Sergeant Miller and his Trauma

Sergeant Miller is a 45-year-old army veteran who attends your clinic for buprenorphine treatment for an opioid use disorder that started with an injury in Afghanistan. He is doing well on the medication, but during a routine follow-up, he mentions he has been having nightmares and avoids crowds. You recognize these as potential symptoms of PTSD. You say, "It sounds like even though you're home, a part of you is still back there. That must be exhausting." You then add, "We know there's a very strong link between traumatic experiences and opioid use. Many veterans find that to really get their life back, they need to treat the trauma as well as the addiction. We have a therapist here who specializes in that. Would you be open to just having a conversation with her?" You have used your knowledge of co-occurring disorders to identify a need and facilitate a warm handoff, addressing the root cause of his substance use.

A Perspective on Wholeness

There is a reason the healthcare system so often separates the mind from the body, and mental health from substance use. It is simpler that way. It allows for neat little boxes and straightforward protocols. But our patients are not simple, and they do not live in boxes. They are whole, complex human beings whose lives are a messy, interwoven story of biology, psychology, and social circumstance. The challenge of co-occurring disorders is a call for nursing to be what it has always been at its best: a profession that refuses to see a person as a diagnosis and insists, instead, on caring for the whole person. Your greatest tool in this work is your holistic perspective.

Key Takeaways for Your Practice

- Assume that your patient with a substance use disorder has a co-occurring mental health condition until proven otherwise, and vice versa.

- Use validated screening tools for both substance use (AUDIT, DAST) and common mental health conditions (PHQ-9, GAD-7) as part of your routine assessment.

- Advocate for integrated treatment plans that address both conditions simultaneously. The old, sequential model of care is ineffective.

- Act as the communication hub between different providers to ensure the patient receives seamless, coordinated care.

Chapter 8: Deconstructing Stigma and Bias in Healthcare

You are in the breakroom, finally getting a chance to sit down, when a colleague walks in, fresh from discharging a patient you both know—a young man with a severe alcohol use disorder who was admitted for the third time this year for pancreatitis. Your colleague sighs, rolls her eyes, and says to the room at large, "Another frequent flyer. He'll be back next month. Some people just don't want to change." A few people nod. Others look down at their phones. An uncomfortable silence hangs in the air. This moment, and thousands like it that happen every day in our healthcare systems, is where stigma lives and breathes. It is the invisible toxin that contaminates our care, undermines our best efforts, and tells our patients that they are not worthy of our help. This chapter is about confronting that toxin head-on.

The Anatomy of Stigma

Stigma is not just about hurt feelings. It is a powerful social force that has measurable, detrimental effects on health. It is a core reason why only a fraction of the people who need treatment for a substance use disorder ever receive it. We can break it down into three interconnected types:

1. **Public Stigma:** This is the collection of negative attitudes and beliefs held by the general population. It is the stereotype of the "junkie" or the "drunk"—the belief that people with substance use disorders are dangerous, weak-willed, and morally flawed. This societal prejudice fuels discrimination in housing, employment, and, yes, in healthcare.

2. **Self-Stigma:** This is what happens when a person internalizes those negative public beliefs. They begin to believe that they *are* weak, flawed, and unworthy of help. This internalized shame leads to secrecy, isolation, and a profound reluctance to seek care for fear of being judged.

3. **Institutional Stigma:** This is when the negative stereotypes are woven into the very fabric of our systems. It can be

explicit—like policies that deny services—or implicit, manifesting as a collective culture of substandard care for a particular group of patients. The eye-rolling in the breakroom is a symptom of institutional stigma. So is the tendency to undertreat the pain of a person with a history of opioid use disorder or to spend less time on patient education with someone we have written off as "non-compliant."

The Uncomfortable Work: Looking in the Mirror

It is easy to point the finger at society or "the system." The more difficult—and more important—work is to turn the lens inward. We all carry biases. We are all products of a society steeped in public stigma. We cannot effectively fight stigma out there until we are willing to confront it in here. This requires a moment of radical honesty.

Ask yourself these questions, and answer them without judgment:

- When you see a patient with track marks on their arms, what is your first, unfiltered thought?

- What messages—spoken or unspoken—did you receive about alcohol and drug use growing up in your family and community?

- Do you find yourself spending less time with, or explaining things less thoroughly to, patients you perceive as "difficult" or "unmotivated"?

- Have you ever used or laughed at terms like "frequent flyer," "addict," or "drug-seeker" in conversation with colleagues?

The goal of this self-reflection is not to induce guilt. Guilt is paralyzing. The goal is to cultivate **awareness**. You cannot change a bias you are unwilling to acknowledge. Awareness is the first step toward consciously choosing a different response—a response grounded in professionalism, empathy, and science.

Practical Strategies for Combating Stigma

Awareness is necessary, but it is not sufficient. You must translate that awareness into action. Here are concrete strategies you can implement today to create a non-judgmental, therapeutically effective clinical environment.

- **Master Person-First Language:** As we discussed in Chapter 1, this is non-negotiable. It is the single most powerful and immediate tool you have. Correct yourself. Gently correct your colleagues. Make it the standard language on your unit. When you consistently say "a person with a substance use disorder," you are actively remodeling the thoughts of those around you.

- **Practice Cultural Humility:** Stigma is often layered with racial, ethnic, and class biases. Cultural humility is the understanding that you are not the expert on anyone else's experience. Approach every patient with genuine curiosity. Ask questions like, "Is there anything about your background or your beliefs that would be helpful for me to know as I care for you?"

- **Advocate in the Moment:** When you see stigma in action— like a patient's report of pain being dismissed—you have a professional obligation to speak up. You do not have to be confrontational. You can be an advocate by using objective, clinical language. "I know this patient has a history of substance use, but his vital signs are elevated, he is guarding his abdomen, and he is rating his pain as a 9/10. He needs a thorough assessment."

- **Challenge Your Colleagues with Compassion:** Addressing the breakroom conversation is delicate. A direct confrontation might backfire. Instead, try pulling the colleague aside later. "You know, that case with Mr. Smith sounded really frustrating. It's tough when we see people struggling so much. I've been reading about how much the brain changes with long-term alcohol use, and it really makes it hard for people to stop, even when they want to." This approach validates your colleague's frustration while gently introducing a more scientific and less moralistic perspective.

Case Examples in Practice

Case Example 1: The Pregnant Patient

A nurse named Sarah is caring for a 22-year-old pregnant woman who has a positive urine screen for cocaine. Sarah's initial, unexamined thought is, "How could she do this to her baby?" She feels a wave of anger and judgment. But then she pauses. She takes a breath and consciously decides to shift her perspective. She walks into the room, sits down, and says, "There is a lot going on right now. How are you doing with all of this?" The young woman bursts into tears and shares a story of trauma and fear. By choosing compassion over condemnation, Sarah opens the door to a real therapeutic connection and is able to connect the patient with prenatal care and substance use treatment.

Case Example 2: The Pain Medication Debate

An elderly man with metastatic cancer and a long-distant history of heroin use is in excruciating pain. The medical resident is hesitant to increase his morphine dose, muttering about the "risk of relapse." The nurse, Maria, steps in. She says to the resident, "Let's focus on the patient's reported goal, which is to be comfortable enough to visit with his grandchildren. His pain is currently preventing that. He has a right to have his pain managed effectively, regardless of his history from 40 years ago. Let's treat the patient in front of us." Her professional, patient-centered advocacy ensures the patient receives the compassionate palliative care he deserves.

Case Example 3: Changing the Unit Culture

An emergency department nurse, Tom, makes a personal commitment to de-stigmatize care. He starts by meticulously using person-first language in his charting and his verbal reports. When a patient who has experienced a non-fatal overdose is successfully revived with naloxone, instead of sighing with exasperation, he says to the team, "Great work, everyone. We saved a life." He makes a point of ensuring every patient with a substance use disorder is offered a referral and a naloxone kit before discharge. Slowly, over months, he notices a change. His colleagues start adopting his language. The "us vs. them" attitude begins to soften. His consistent, professional modeling has begun to shift the entire unit's culture.

Chapter 9: Trauma-Informed Care

Asking "What Happened to You?"

We can not talk about addiction without talking about trauma. The two are inextricably linked. For an enormous number of people struggling with a substance use disorder, the substance use did not start as a party or a bad decision. It started as a solution. It was a desperate attempt to numb the pain, quiet the intrusive memories, or escape the crushing anxiety left in the wake of a traumatic experience. If we as nurses only treat the substance use without acknowledging the underlying wound, we are, at best, placing a small bandage on a raging infection. To provide truly effective care, we must shift our fundamental question from, "What's wrong with you?" to the far more compassionate and useful question, "What happened to you?" This is the essence of Trauma-Informed Care.

What Trauma-Informed Care Is—And Is Not

Let's be very clear. Trauma-Informed Care (TIC) is **not** about you becoming a trauma therapist. It does not mean you are expected to conduct intensive psychotherapy sessions at the bedside. Rather, TIC is an organizational and clinical framework that involves:

- **Realizing** the widespread impact of trauma and understanding potential paths for recovery.

- **Recognizing** the signs and symptoms of trauma in patients, families, and staff.

- **Responding** by fully integrating knowledge about trauma into policies, procedures, and practices.

- **Resisting Re-traumatization** by creating a care environment that is safe and empowering.

Think of it as applying universal precautions for psychological safety. We create environments that are safe for everyone, because we operate under the assumption that anyone we care for could have a history of trauma.

The Brain on Trauma: A Survival Mechanism

To understand why trauma and addiction are so linked, we need to understand a little about the brain. A traumatic event—a situation that overwhelms a person's ability to cope—throws the brain's stress response system into overdrive. The amygdala, the brain's "smoke detector," becomes hyper-vigilant, constantly scanning for danger. The body is flooded with stress hormones like cortisol and adrenaline. This "fight, flight, or freeze" response is a brilliant survival mechanism in the short term. But for someone with post-traumatic stress, that alarm system gets stuck in the "on" position. They may live in a state of constant physiological arousal, anxiety, and fear.

Now, consider the effects of substances we have discussed. Opioids numb all pain, physical and emotional. Alcohol depresses the over-active central nervous system. Benzodiazepines quiet the unrelenting anxiety. From the perspective of a dysregulated nervous system, these substances can feel like medicine. They offer a temporary—but powerful—respite from the internal storm of trauma.

The Five Principles of TIC in Your Daily Practice

Applying TIC is about making small, intentional changes in how you interact with every patient. Here are the five core principles and how you can apply them.

1. **Safety:** Your first priority is to create an environment of both physical and psychological safety.

   o **Practical Steps:** Knock on the door and wait for a response. Introduce yourself and your role every time you enter. Ask for permission before touching a patient ("Is it okay if I check your blood pressure now?"). Pull the curtain for privacy. Explain noises and procedures before they happen to avoid surprises.

2. **Trustworthiness and Transparency:** Trust is often shattered by trauma. Your job is to be reliable, consistent, and honest.

- **Practical Steps:** Do what you say you will do. If you promise to come back with a blanket, come back with the blanket. If a procedure is going to be painful, be honest about it while also reassuring them you will do everything you can to make it as comfortable as possible.

3. **Choice:** Trauma often involves a profound loss of control. Restoring a sense of choice, even in small ways, can be incredibly empowering.

   - **Practical Steps:** Offer simple choices whenever possible. "Would you prefer to sit in the chair or on the bed?" "I need to draw some blood. Which arm would you prefer I use?" "Would you like a family member to be with you for this conversation?"

4. **Collaboration and Mutuality:** Level the power dynamic. Move from doing things *to* a patient to doing things *with* a patient.

   - **Practical Steps:** Use the language of partnership. "Let's work together on a plan to manage your pain." Ask for their input. "You are the expert on your own body. What has worked for you in the past?"

5. **Empowerment and Strengths:** See beyond the trauma and the diagnosis to the person's inherent strengths and resilience.

   - **Practical Steps:** Use affirmations that recognize their strength. "The fact that you are here seeking help after everything you have been through is a testament to your courage." Help them identify their own coping skills. "What is one thing that helps you feel even a little bit calmer when you get overwhelmed?"

Case Examples in Practice

Case Example 1: The Modified Exam

A patient named Elena discloses to her primary care nurse that she is a survivor of sexual assault. She is due for a pelvic exam, which she has been avoiding for years out of fear. The nurse, applying TIC principles, completely changes the approach. She sits down with Elena first, in her street clothes, to discuss the exam. She explains every single step of what will happen. She assures Elena that she can say "stop" at any time, for any reason. During the exam, she positions herself at Elena's side, not at the foot of the bed, and continues to explain everything she is doing *before* she does it. By prioritizing safety, transparency, and choice, the nurse helps Elena complete a necessary health screening in a way that feels empowering rather than re-traumatizing.

Case Example 2: The Agitated Veteran

A veteran on an inpatient psychiatric unit becomes highly agitated every time the meal cart is wheeled down the hall, with its loud, clanging noises. The staff has labeled him as "disruptive." A trauma-informed nurse, however, hypothesizes that the noise might be a trigger for his combat-related PTSD. Instead of punishing the behavior, she collaborates with the patient. "I've noticed that the noise in the hallway seems to be really difficult for you. I'm wondering if you'd prefer to take your meals in the quiet room at the end of the hall?" The veteran agrees, and his "disruptive" behavior ceases. The nurse has correctly identified a trauma trigger and modified the environment to enhance the patient's sense of safety.

Case Example 3: Building Trust with a Quiet Patient

A home health nurse is visiting a new patient, a middle-aged man with severe diabetes who rarely speaks and avoids eye contact. Previous nurses have described him as "uncooperative." The new nurse, suspecting a possible trauma history, decides to focus solely on building trust. For the first few visits, she is simply predictable and consistent. She arrives exactly on time. She performs her tasks efficiently and quietly, explaining each step. She never pushes him to talk but creates a calm, safe presence. On the fourth visit, as she is packing up her bag, the patient quietly says, "No one ever treated me nice when I was a kid." This small disclosure is a monumental step, made possible only because the nurse first built a foundation of safety and trust.

Chapter 10: The Harm Reduction Philosophy in Practice

We have now arrived at what may be one of the most misunderstood—and most important—concepts in modern addiction care: harm reduction. For some, the idea of harm reduction is controversial. It can feel like we are "enabling" or "condoning" drug use. This comes from a place of all-or-nothing thinking, a belief that total, immediate abstinence is the only acceptable outcome. But what about the patient who is not ready, or able, to stop using right now? Do we turn our backs on them? Or do we meet them exactly where they are, with a set of practical, life-saving strategies? Harm reduction chooses the latter. It is a philosophy rooted in pragmatism, public health, and radical compassion. It is the belief that every human life is valuable and worthy of care, right here, right now.

The Core of the Philosophy

Harm reduction is a set of practical strategies and ideas aimed at reducing the negative consequences associated with drug use. It is also a social justice movement built on a belief in—and respect for—the rights of people who use drugs. Its core principles include:

- **Accepting that drug use is a part of our world** and choosing to work to minimize its harmful effects rather than simply ignore or condemn them.

- **Meeting people "where they're at"** and not judging them for where they are on their journey.

- **Empowering people who use drugs** as the primary agents of reducing the harms of their own drug use.

- **Prioritizing human life and dignity** over a single, narrow definition of "recovery."

As a nurse, embracing harm reduction means accepting that you can care for someone and work to keep them safe, even if you do not agree with their choices. It means focusing on *any positive change*.

The Nurse's Role in Practical Harm Reduction

This is not just abstract philosophy. It involves specific, actionable nursing interventions that you can—and should—be providing.

Overdose Prevention and Naloxone Education

This is perhaps the most critical harm reduction strategy in the era of fentanyl. Every person at risk of an opioid overdose, and their family and friends, should have a naloxone kit and know how to use it. You are the perfect person to provide this training. It can be done in less than five minutes.

A Step-by-Step Guide to Naloxone Training:

1. **Recognize the Overdose:** Teach the simple signs. A person who is not responding to shouting or a sternal rub, has slow or no breathing, blue lips, and pinpoint pupils.

2. **Call for Help:** The first step is always to call 911.

3. **Administer Naloxone:** Show them how to use the specific device you are dispensing (nasal spray is most common). "Peel back the package. Place the tip in one nostril. Press the plunger firmly. It's that simple."

4. **Perform Rescue Breathing:** Explain that the naloxone can take a minute or two to work, but the brain needs oxygen *now*. Teach them to tilt the head back, make a seal over the mouth, and give one breath every five seconds.

5. **Stay and Support:** Explain that naloxone wears off in 30-90 minutes, but the opioids can last much longer. The person can go back into an overdose. It is essential to stay with them until help arrives.

Safer Use Education

This can feel like the most challenging part, but it is also one of the most important. You are providing people with information to keep themselves alive. This must be done without judgment.

- **For Injection Drug Use:** "Using a new, sterile syringe every single time is the best way to prevent infections like HIV and Hepatitis C. It also helps prevent abscesses and other skin infections."

- **For Preventing Overdose:** "Fentanyl is in almost everything now. It's much safer if you don't use alone. If you must use alone, could you have a friend you trust check in on you? Another strategy is to 'test your shot' by only using a small amount first to see how strong it is."

- **For Pill or Powder Use:** "Using your own supplies—like straws or pipes—and not sharing them can prevent the spread of infections."

Connecting to Harm Reduction Services

You must know the resources in your community. Your role is often to be the bridge between the formal healthcare system and these essential community-based programs.

- **Syringe Service Programs (SSPs):** These are places where people can get sterile injection equipment, dispose of used syringes safely, and often access other services like wound care, infectious disease testing, and referrals to treatment.

- **Safe Consumption Sites (SCS) / Overdose Prevention Centers (OPCs):** Where legal, these are facilities where people can use pre-obtained drugs in a clean, safe environment, supervised by trained staff who can intervene in the event of an overdose.

Referring a patient to these services is a powerful act of care. It tells them you are invested in their survival and well-being, no matter what.

Case Examples in Practice

Case Example 1: The ED Discharge

A young man is treated in the emergency department for a non-fatal opioid overdose. After he is stabilized, the discharging nurse, Anna, does not just give him a pamphlet. She sits with him and his brother. She says, "That was incredibly scary, and I am so glad you are okay. I want to give you a tool that can prevent this from happening again." She pulls out a naloxone kit, demonstrates how to use it, and has his brother repeat the instructions back to her. She provides two kits— one for the patient and one for the brother. This five-minute intervention has dramatically increased the safety of that entire household.

Case Example 2: The Wound Care Visit

A street nurse is providing wound care for a woman who is experiencing homelessness and who injects heroin. While cleaning and dressing a large abscess on her arm, the nurse says, in a matter-of-fact tone, "It looks like you're having a hard time finding clean spots. I have some new syringes here for you if you need them. Also, the community health van is on the next block. They have a nurse who can help you check for infections." The nurse has used the opportunity of treating a complication of drug use to also provide tools and resources to prevent future complications.

Case Example 3: A Primary Care Conversation

During a routine visit, a patient mentions to his primary care nurse that his son is actively using fentanyl. The patient is terrified. The nurse validates his fear, saying, "That sounds incredibly stressful. It makes sense that you are worried." Then, she pivots to empowerment. "While you can't control your son's use, there are things you can do to keep him safer. One of the most important is having naloxone in the house. Let me get you a kit and show you how to use it. It's like having a fire extinguisher. You hope you never need it, but if you do, it can save a life." She has given this father a concrete, positive action he can take in the face of a terrifying and seemingly powerless situation.

A Final Charge

Throughout this book, we have traveled from the inner workings of the brain to the outer edges of our communities. We have examined the science of pharmacology, the structure of a care plan, and the art of a therapeutic conversation. We have confronted the shadows of stigma and the ghosts of trauma. If there is one single thread that ties all of this together, it is this: your presence matters. The knowledge you have gained is a set of tools, but the true instrument of healing is you. It is the steady, compassionate, non-judgmental presence you bring to the bedside, the clinic, or the street outreach van.

You will have days when you feel frustrated. You will care for people who return to use. You will witness immense suffering. But you will also see moments of breathtaking courage. You will hold the hand of someone starting a new medication and a new life. You will teach a mother how to save her son's life with naloxone. You will be the first person in a patient's entire life to ask, "What happened to you?" and truly listen to the answer.

This work is not easy. But it is, without question, some of the most important and rewarding work a nurse can do. Never doubt your ability to be a powerful force for healing, for safety, and for hope. You are the lighthouse in the storm. Now go, and let your light shine.

Key Takeaways for Your Practice

- Harm reduction is a practical, evidence-based approach that prioritizes keeping people safe and alive.

- Teaching patients and families how to recognize an overdose and use naloxone is a core nursing function.

- Providing non-judgmental education on safer use practices is an effective strategy to reduce infections and other harms.

- Know and confidently refer to the harm reduction resources in your community, like syringe service programs.

Chapter 11: Case Studies from the Front Lines

Theory is a map. It is essential for understanding the terrain, for planning a route, and for knowing what to expect. But a map is not the journey itself. The real work of nursing happens on the ground, in the messy, unpredictable, and profoundly human interactions with our patients. This final chapter is the clinical rotation for this book. Here, we will take the maps we have drawn in the preceding chapters—the science of addiction, the models of care, the communication skills—and apply them to the real world. We will follow four patients through four different settings, demonstrating how you can integrate these concepts into a seamless, compassionate, and effective nursing practice.

Case 1: The Emergency Department—An Overdose, An Opening

The Situation

Liam, a 24-year-old man, is brought into the Emergency Department by paramedics. He was found unresponsive in a coffee shop bathroom by a friend. On arrival, he is cyanotic, with a respiratory rate of 6 breaths per minute and pupils constricted to pinpoints. His friend, frantic, says Liam has been using heroin.

The Nursing Response

You are the primary nurse, and your first actions are automatic, grounded in the ABCs—Airway, Breathing, Circulation.

1. **Stabilization:** You immediately apply a non-rebreather mask at 15 liters per minute while another nurse establishes IV access. You connect him to the cardiac monitor and pulse oximeter. His oxygen saturation is 82%. You know that every second counts.

2. **Naloxone Administration:** The physician orders 0.4 mg of naloxone IV push. You administer the dose swiftly. There is no immediate response. You know that with the prevalence of fentanyl, higher doses are often needed. After a minute, a second dose of 1 mg is ordered and given.

3. **The Revival and the Aftermath (Trauma-Informed Care):** About 45 seconds after the second dose, Liam gasps. His eyes fly open, and he sits up, immediately trying to pull off his oxygen mask. He is confused, agitated, and sweating. His first words are a curse. You recognize this is not aggression; it is the violent shock of sudden, precipitated withdrawal. You lower your own voice and your posture, making sure not to stand over him. "Liam, my name is Chris. You're in the hospital. You had an overdose. We gave you a medicine to help you breathe. I know you feel terrible right now. You are safe." You have applied the TIC principles of **Safety** and **Transparency**.

4. **Engaging with Motivational Interviewing:** Once Liam is calmer and more oriented, you find a moment of quiet. You pull up a stool to sit at his level.

   - **You (Open Question):** "That was a really scary experience. What's going through your mind right now?"

   - **Liam:** "I can't believe this happened. My friend must think I'm a total loser."

   - **You (Complex Reflection):** "It sounds like you're less worried about what happened and more worried about how this affects your relationships and what people think of you."

   - **Liam:** "Yeah... I just... I don't want to be *that guy*."

   - **You (Affirmation):** "The fact that you're thinking about that right now tells me that your friendships are really important to you."

5. **Brief Intervention:** You see an opening.

   - **You:** "Liam, would it be okay if I shared what happens from a medical standpoint when someone overdoses? It might help make sense of what just happened."

70

(Asking **Permission**). Liam shrugs, a sign of assent. You briefly explain how opioids suppress the drive to breathe. You link it directly to his experience. "That's why you were turning blue when you came in. It was a very close call." (Providing **Feedback**).

- ○ **You:** "Where does this leave you now?" (Eliciting a **Response**).

- ○ **Liam:** "I don't know. I can't keep doing this."

6. **The Warm Handoff (Referral to Treatment):** You recognize this flicker of "change talk." Your hospital has a peer recovery coach program.

   - ○ **You:** "Liam, we have people on our team who have been through this themselves. They're called recovery coaches. They know what it's like, and they know how to find help. Would you be open to talking to one of them before you leave? His name is Mike."

   - ○ Liam nods. You page Mike, who comes to the ED. You introduce them: "Liam, this is Mike, the peer recovery coach I was telling you about. Mike, this is Liam." You have now facilitated a warm handoff, connecting Liam to a person, not just a system.

Case 2: The Medical-Surgical Floor—Withdrawal and Pain

The Situation

Brenda is a 55-year-old woman admitted for a laparoscopic cholecystectomy. During her intake, she tells you she drinks "a few glasses of wine" every night. You, however, ask the AUDIT questions and her score is 19, indicating harmful use. It is now 48 hours after her surgery and her last drink. You walk into her room and she is tremulous, diaphoretic, and her heart rate is 118 bpm.

The Nursing Response

You have anticipated this. Your proactive screening on admission prepared you for the possibility of alcohol withdrawal.

1. **Objective Assessment:** You immediately grab a CIWA-Ar flowsheet. You sit with Brenda and systematically score her symptoms. She reports nausea, her hands have a noticeable tremor, and she seems intensely anxious and sensitive to the light. Her total score is 16.

2. **Implementing the Care Plan:** You have a standing order set for withdrawal management.

   - **Pharmacological Intervention:** Based on her score of 16, the protocol calls for 2 mg of lorazepam. You administer the medication and document it on the flowsheet. You tell Brenda, "Brenda, your body is going through a reaction from the lack of alcohol. This medication will help calm your nervous system and keep you safe. I'll be checking on you very frequently."

   - **Non-Pharmacological Intervention:** You dim the lights in her room, turn off the television, and bring her a cool cloth for her forehead. You have addressed the **Risk for Injury** by creating a low-stimulus environment.

3. **Navigating Pain Management:** Brenda is also reporting 7/10 surgical pain. She is due for her PRN oxycodone. You know that managing post-op pain in a patient with a substance use disorder can be complex. You formulate a plan.

   - **Advocacy:** You call the surgical resident. "This is Sarah, Brenda Smith's nurse. I've just given her lorazepam for a CIWA score of 16. She is also reporting 7/10 incisional pain. I'm concerned about relying solely on opioids for her pain, given the risk of over-sedation when combined with the benzodiazepine. I'd like to suggest we start scheduled acetaminophen and ibuprofen to provide a baseline of non-opioid analgesia. Can we get an order for that?"

- ○ **Patient Education:** You explain the multi-modal pain plan to Brenda. "Brenda, we're going to give you your prescribed oxycodone for the surgical pain. We're also going to start some other non-opioid pain relievers to attack the pain from a different angle. This should give you better relief and keep you safer." You have addressed her pain while also prioritizing her safety.

Case 3: The Primary Care Clinic—A Routine Visit, A Pivotal Conversation

The Situation

David, a 45-year-old man, is at your clinic for his annual physical. He has a history of hypertension and type 2 diabetes, both of which are poorly controlled. As part of the standard rooming process, you ask him the AUDIT questions. He seems surprised but answers them. His score is 14.

The Nursing Response

You recognize this as a critical opportunity to intervene early.

1. **Screening and Feedback:** You finish the rest of the intake. Then, before the physician comes in, you say, "David, thank you for answering those questions about alcohol use. I've tallied your score, and it falls into a range—about 14—that research shows can increase health risks, especially for things like blood pressure and blood sugar control. Would you be willing to talk with me about that for a few minutes?" You have asked **Permission**.

2. **The Brief Intervention:**

- ○ **You (Linking to Health Goals):** "You mentioned earlier that you're frustrated about your blood pressure still being high even with the medication. What you might

73

not know is that drinking at this level can actually work against what the blood pressure medicine is trying to do."

- o **David:** "Really? I thought a little red wine was supposed to be good for you."

- o **You (Providing Information):** "That's a common belief, but the evidence shows that for men, drinking more than four drinks on any day or more than 14 in a week can raise blood pressure. Your score indicates you're a bit above that. What are your thoughts about that?"

- o **David:** "I had no idea. I just... it's how I unwind after work."

- o **You (Summarizing and Exploring Ambivalence):** "So on the one hand, having a few drinks is a really important way for you to de-stress from your day. On the other hand, it might be one of the things getting in the way of you reaching your health goals. That's a tough spot to be in."

3. **Collaborative Goal Setting:**

- o **You:** "I'm not asking you to stop drinking entirely, unless that's what you want. I'm wondering what you would think about an experiment. What if, for the next month, you tried to stick within those low-risk guidelines—no more than four on a day, no more than 14 in a week—and we see what happens to your blood pressure at your follow-up visit?"

- o **David:** "I guess I could try that."

- o You have collaborated on a small, concrete, measurable goal. You have empowered David to take an active role in his own health, all within the space of a 7-minute conversation.

Case 4: The Community Health Setting—A Circle of Care

The Situation

You are a community health nurse. One of your patients is Jasmine, a 28-year-old woman who is 20 weeks pregnant. She has an opioid use disorder and is stable on buprenorphine. She has a history of significant trauma.

The Nursing Response

Your role here is multifaceted: you are an educator, a coordinator, a counselor, and an advocate.

1. **Trauma-Informed and Stigma-Free Care:** At every visit, you make a point of creating a safe and collaborative environment. You know she has appointments at multiple places where she may face judgment. Your office is her safe harbor. You always ask, "How are things going for you? What's been the most stressful part of your week?" You are asking about her life, not just her condition.

2. **Patient Education on MAT:** Jasmine expresses fear that the buprenorphine will harm her baby.

   o **You:** "Jasmine, that is such an important question, and it shows how much you care about this baby. Let me reassure you. Staying on your buprenorphine is the single best thing you can do for you and the baby right now. It keeps you stable and safe, which keeps the baby stable and safe. It dramatically reduces the risk of overdose and other complications. We will have a team ready to care for the baby after birth for any symptoms they might have." You have provided clear, evidence-based, reassuring information.

3. **Harm Reduction Counseling:** You know that a return to use is possible for anyone.

- **You:** "Jasmine, we have a naloxone kit for you today. I want you to have it, and I want your partner to know where it is and how to use it. It's like having a fire extinguisher in the kitchen. You hope you never need it, but it's there to keep you safe just in case." You are planning for safety without judgment.

4. **Care Coordination:** Jasmine is overwhelmed by her appointments. You take out a calendar and a pen.

   - **You:** "Okay, let's map this out. You have your OB appointment on Tuesday, your buprenorphine provider on Wednesday, and your WIC appointment on Friday. I'm going to call your OB provider right now, with you here, just to make sure they have all the right information about your buprenorphine dose so everyone is on the same page." You act as the central hub, ensuring that all the pieces of her fragmented care are connected into a supportive whole.

Appendix: The Nurse's Quick-Reference Toolkit

This section is designed for the real world. These are tools you can photocopy, laminate, and put on your clipboard or download to your phone. They are meant for quick reference at the point of care.

Common Screening Questionnaires

The CAGE Questionnaire

A quick, 4-item screen for alcohol use disorder. Two or more "yes" answers suggest a problem.

- Have you ever felt you should **C**ut down on your drinking?[1]

- Have people **A**nnoyed you by criticizing your drinking?[2]

- Have you ever felt bad or **G**uilty about your drinking?[3]

- Have you ever had a drink first thing in the morning to steady your nerves [4]or get rid of a hangover (**E**ye-opener)?

The AUDIT (Alcohol Use Disorders Identification Test)

(This would be a full, formatted version of the 10-item questionnaire with clear scoring instructions as provided in Chapter 3).

The DAST-10 (Drug Abuse Screening Test)

(This would be a full, formatted version of the 10-item questionnaire with clear scoring instructions as provided in Chapter 3).

Withdrawal Assessment Scales

CIWA-Ar (Clinical Institute Withdrawal Assessment for Alcohol, Revised)

(This section would feature the full scale, with each of the 10 items listed alongside the scoring range, e.g., "Nausea & Vomiting: 0 - None, 1 - Mild nausea, ... 7 - Constant nausea and frequent vomiting." It would also include the scoring thresholds for intervention).

COWS (Clinical Opiate Withdrawal Scale)

(This section would feature the full scale, listing all 11 items and their scoring criteria, along with the final score interpretation: 5-12 Mild, 13-24 Moderate, etc.).

Motivational Interviewing "Cheat Sheet"

Core Spirit: Partnership, Acceptance, Compassion, Evocation (PACE)

Core Skills (OARS):

Skill	Purpose	Example Stems
Open Questions	To invite conversation & exploration	"What are the good things about...?" "Tell me more about..." "How does that affect you?" "What would you like to see happen?"
Affirmations	To recognize strengths & build confidence	"That took a lot of courage to say." "You're clearly a resourceful person." "You've handled a lot." "That's a good point."
Reflections	To show you are listening & understand	**Simple:** "You're feeling..." "It sounds like..." **Complex:** "On the one hand..., and on the

Skill	Purpose	Example Stems
		other..." "You're wondering if..."
Summaries	To recap & transition	"Let me see if I've got this right..." "So, it sounds like the key things for you are..."

Listening for Change Talk (DARN):

- **D**esire: "I want to..." "I wish I could..."
- **A**bility: "I think I could..." "I might be able to..."
- **R**eason: "I would have more energy if..." "It would help my blood pressure..."
- **N**eed: "I have to..." "I must..."

Patient Education Handout Templates

(This section would contain simplified, visually appealing, one-page templates.)

Template 1: What is Buprenorphine (Suboxone)?

- **What it is:** A medication to treat opioid use disorder.
- **How it works:** It quiets cravings and stops withdrawal, helping your brain heal.
- **How to take it:** Let the film dissolve completely under your tongue.
- **Common Side Effects:** Constipation, headache, sweating. (Talk to your nurse about how to manage these!)

- **Key Safety Point:** It is a life-saving medication. Taking it every day is the best thing you can do for your recovery.

Template 2: How to Use Naloxone (Narcan) to Reverse an Overdose

(This would be highly visual, with simple graphics for each step.)

1. **CHECK for Response:** Shout name and rub the middle of their chest hard.

2. **CALL 911:** Tell them someone is not breathing.

3. **GIVE NALOXONE:** Peel package. Place tip in one nostril. Press plunger firmly.

4. **GIVE RESCUE BREATHS:** One breath every 5 seconds.

5. **STAY WITH THEM** until help arrives. If they don't wake up in 2-3 minutes, give the second dose.

Glossary of Common Terms and Acronyms

- **Agonist:** A substance that activates a receptor in the brain. (e.g., heroin, methadone).

- **Antagonist:** A substance that blocks a receptor in the brain. (e.g., naltrexone, naloxone).

- **AUDIT:** Alcohol Use Disorders Identification Test.

- **CIWA-Ar:** Clinical Institute Withdrawal Assessment for Alcohol, Revised.

- **COWS:** Clinical Opiate Withdrawal Scale.

- **DAST:** Drug Abuse Screening Test.

- **Harm Reduction:** Policies and strategies aimed at reducing the negative consequences of substance use.[5]

- **MAT:** Medication-Assisted Treatment.

- **MOUD:** Medications for Opioid Use Disorder (the preferred term for MAT for opioids).

- **Partial Agonist:** A substance that only partially activates a receptor.[6] (e.g., buprenorphine).

- **SBIRT:** Screening, Brief Intervention, and Referral to Treatment.

- **TIC:** Trauma-Informed Care.

A Final Word

We have reached the end of our journey through this guide, but we have only reached the beginning of yours. The knowledge and skills contained in these pages are not meant to sit on a shelf. They are meant to be used, to be adapted, to be integrated into the unique art and science of your own nursing practice. This work is a profound challenge, but it is also a profound privilege. To be the person who offers a hand to someone in the deepest despair, to be the one who provides safety in a moment of chaos, to be the voice of science and compassion in a world filled with stigma—this is the very heart of nursing. Go forward with confidence, with curiosity, and with the unwavering belief in the capacity of every person to heal.

References

[1] Maté, G. (2008). *In the Realm of Hungry Ghosts: Close Encounters with Addiction*.[7] Knopf Canada.

[2] University of Pittsburgh School of Nursing. (n.d.). *SBIRT for Undergraduate Nursing Students*. Retrieved from https://www.nursing.pitt.edu/continuing-ed/sbirt-teaching-resources/undergraduate-students

[3] Miller, W. R., & Rollnick, S. (2013). *Motivational Interviewing: Helping People Change* (3rd ed.). The Guilford Press.[8]

[4] Dart, M. A. (2011). *Motivational Interviewing in Nursing Practice: Empowering the Patient*. Jones & Bartlett Learning.

[5] Substance Abuse and Mental Health Services Administration. (2014). *SAMHSA's Concept of Trauma and Guidance for a Trauma-Informed Approach*. HHS Publication No. (SMA) 14-4884.

[6] Harm Reduction Coalition. (n.d.). *Principles of Harm Reduction*. Retrieved from https://harmreduction.org/about-us/principles-of-harm-reduction/